# Ultimate Keto Chaffles Cooking Guide

*Innovative and Delicious Chaffle Ideas for Any Occasion*

*Imogene Cook*

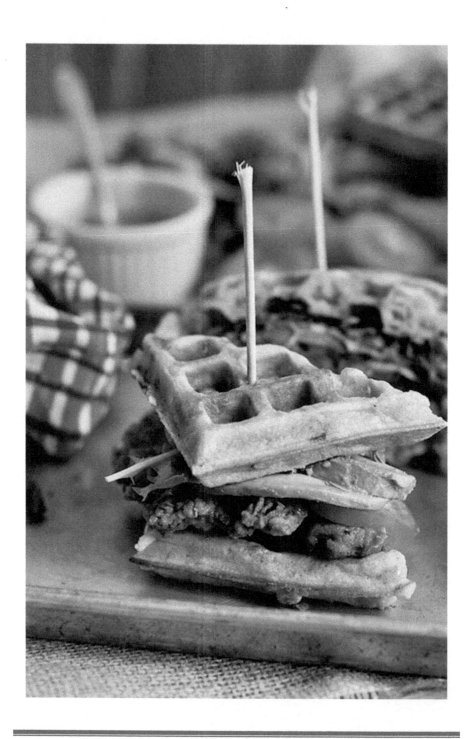

# TABLE OF CONTENTS

# How to Make Chaffles?

## Equipment and Ingredients Discussed

Making chaffles requires five simple steps and nothing more than a waffle maker for flat chaffles and a waffle bowl maker for chaffle bowls.

To make chaffles, you will need two necessary ingredients —eggs and cheese. My preferred cheeses are cheddar cheese or mozzarella cheese. These melt quickly, making them the go-to for most recipes. Meanwhile, always ensure that your cheeses are finely grated or thinly sliced for use.

Now, to make a standard chaffle:

First, preheat your waffle maker until adequately hot.

Meanwhile, in a bowl, mix the egg with cheese on hand until well combined.

Open the iron, pour in a quarter or half of the mixture, and close.

Cook the chaffle for 5 to 7 minutes or until it is crispy.

Transfer the chaffle to a plate and allow cooling before serving.

# 11 Tips to Make Chaffles

My surefire ways to turn out the crispiest of chaffles:

**Preheat Well:** Yes! It sounds obvious to preheat the waffle iron before usage. However, preheating the iron moderately

will not get your chaffles as crispy as you will like. The best way to preheat before cooking is to ensure that the iron is very hot.

**Not-So-Cheesy:** Will you prefer to have your chaffles less cheesy? Then use mozzarella cheese.

**Not-So Eggy:** If you aren't comfortable with the smell of eggs in your chaffles, try using egg whites instead of egg yolks or whole eggs.

**To Shred or to Slice:** Many recipes call for shredded cheese when making chaffles, but I find sliced cheeses to offer crispier pieces. While I stick with mostly shredded cheese for convenience's sake, be at ease to use sliced cheese in the same quantity. When using sliced cheeses, arrange two to four pieces in the waffle iron, top with the beaten eggs, and some slices of the cheese. Cover and cook until crispy.

**Shallower Irons:** For better crisps on your chaffles, use shallower waffle irons as they cook easier and faster.

**Layering:** Don't fill up the waffle iron with too much batter. Work between a quarter and a half cup of total ingredients per batch for correctly done chaffles.

**Patience:** It is a virtue even when making chaffles. For the best results, allow the chaffles to sit in the iron for 5 to 7 minutes before serving.

**No Peeking:** 7 minutes isn't too much of a time to wait for the outcome of your chaffles, in my opinion.

Opening the iron and checking on the chaffle before

it is done stands you a worse chance of ruining it.

**Crispy Cooling:** For better crisp, I find that allowing the chaffles to cool further after they are transferred to a plate aids a lot.

**Easy Cleaning:** For the best cleanup, wet a paper towel and wipe the inner parts of the iron clean while still warm. Kindly note that the iron should be warm but not hot!

**Brush It:** Also, use a clean toothbrush to clean between the iron's teeth for a thorough cleanup. You may also use a dry, rough sponge to clean the iron while it is still warm.

# Parmesan Garlic Chaffle

Preparation time: 6 minutes

Cooking Time: 5 Minutes

Servings: 2

## Ingredients:

- 1 Tbsp fresh garlic minced
- 2 Tbsp butter
- 1-oz cream cheese, cubed
- 2 Tbsp almond flour
- 1 tsp baking soda
- 2 large eggs
- 1 tsp dried chives
- ½ cup parmesan cheese, shredded
- ¾ cup mozzarella cheese, shredded

## Directions:

1. Heat cream cheese and butter in a saucepan over medium-low until melted.
2. Add garlic and cook, stirring, for minutes.

3. Turn on waffle maker to heat and oil it with cooking spray.
4. In a small mixing bowl, whisk together flour and baking soda, then set aside.
5. In a separate bowl, beat eggs for 1 minute 30 seconds on high, then add in cream cheese mixture and beat for 60 seconds more.
6. Add flour mixture, chives, and cheeses to the bowl and stir well.
7. Add ¼ cup batter to waffle maker.
8. Close and cook for 4 minutes, until golden brown.
9. Repeat for remaining batter.
10. Add favorite toppings and serve.

**Nutrition:**

Carbs: 5 g ; Fat: 33 g ; Protein: 19 g ; Calories: 385

# Chicken & Veggies Chaffles

Preparation time: 10 minutes

Cooking Time: 15 Minutes

Servings: 2

## Ingredients:

- 1/3 cup cooked grass-fed chicken, chopped
- 1/3 cup cooked spinach, chopped
- 1/3 cup marinated artichokes, chopped
- 1 organic egg, beaten
- 1/3 cup Mozzarella cheese, shredded
- 1 ounce cream cheese, softened
- ¼ teaspoon garlic powder

## Directions:

1. Preheat a mini waffle iron and then grease it.
2. In a medium bowl, place all ingredients and mix until well combined.
3. Place 1/of the mixture into preheated waffle iron and cook for about 4-5 minutes or until golden brown.

4. Repeat with the remaining mixture.

5. Serve warm.

## Nutrition:

Calories:95  Net  Carb:1.3g  Fat:5.8g  Saturated  Fat:1.3g Carbohydrates: 2.2g Dietary Fiber: 0.9g Sugar: 0.3g Protein: 8.

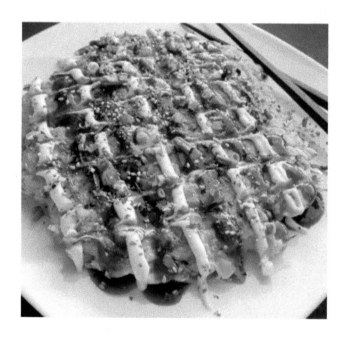

# Turkey Chaffles

Preparation time: 10 minutes

Cooking Time: 16 Minutes

Servings: 2

## Ingredients:

- ½ cup cooked turkey meat, chopped
- 2 organic eggs, beaten
- ½ cup Parmesan cheese, grated
- ½ cup Mozzarella, shredded
- ¼ teaspoon poultry seasoning
- ¼ teaspoon onion powder

## Directions:

1. Preheat a mini waffle iron and then grease it.
2. In a medium bowl, place all ingredients and mix until well combined.
3. Place ¼ of the mixture into preheated waffle iron and cook for about 4 minutes or until golden brown.
4. Repeat with the remaining mixture.

5. Serve warm.

## Nutrition:

Calories:108    Net    Carb:0.5g    Fat:1g    Saturated    Fat:2.6g
Carbohydrates: 0.5g Dietary Fiber: 0g Sugar: 0.2g Protein: 12.9g

# Chicken & Zucchini Chaffles

Servings: 9

Cooking Time: 0 Minutes

## Ingredients:

- 4 ounces cooked grass-fed chicken, chopped
- 2 cups zucchini, shredded and squeezed
- ¼ cup scallion, chopped
- 2 large organic eggs
- ½ cup Mozzarella cheese, shredded
- ½ cup Cheddar cheese, shredded
- ½ cup blanched almond flour
- 1 teaspoon organic baking powder
- ½ teaspoon garlic salt
- ½ teaspoon onion powder

## Directions:

1. Preheat a waffle iron and then grease it.
2. In a medium bowl, place all ingredients and mix until well combined.

3. Divide the mixture into 9 portions.
4. Place 1 portion of the mixture into preheated waffle iron and cook for about 2-3 minutes or until golden brown.
5. Repeat with the remaining mixture.
6. Serve warm.

## Nutrition:

Calories:108   Net   Carb:2g   Fat:6.9g   Saturated   Fat:2.2g Carbohydrates: 3.1g Dietary Fiber: 1.1g Sugar: 0. Protein: 8.8g

# Pepperoni Chaffles

Preparation time: 5 minutes

Cooking Time: 5 Minutes

Servings: 2

## Ingredients:

- 1 organic egg, beaten
- ½ cup Mozzarella cheese, shredded
- 2 tablespoons turkey pepperoni slice, chopped
- 1 tablespoon sugar-free pizza sauce
- ¼ teaspoon Italian seasoning

## Directions:

1. Preheat a waffle iron and then grease it.
2. In a bowl, place all the ingredients and mix well.
3. Place the mixture into preheated waffle iron and cook for about 5 minutes or until golden brown.
4. Serve warm.

**Nutrition:**

Calories:119    Net    Carb:2.4g    Fat:7.g    Saturated    Fat:3g
Carbohydrates: 2.7g Dietary Fiber: 0.3g Sugar: 0.9g Protein:
10.3g

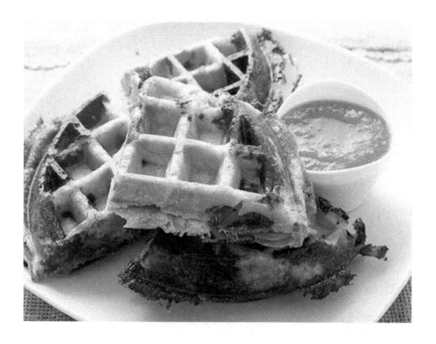

# Hot Sauce Jalapeño Chaffles

Preparation time: 6 minutes

Cooking Time: 8 Minutes

Servings: 2

## Ingredients:

- ½ cup plus 2 teaspoons Cheddar cheese, shredded and divided
- 1 organic egg, beaten
- 6 jalapeño pepper slices
- ¼ teaspoon hot sauce
- Pinch of salt

## Directions:

1. Preheat a mini waffle iron and then grease it.
2. In a bowl, place ½ cup of cheese and remaining ingredients and mix until well combined.
3. Place about 1 teaspoon of cheese in the bottom of the waffle maker for about seconds before adding the mixture.

4. Place half of the mixture into preheated waffle iron and cook for about 3-minutes or until golden brown.
5. Repeat with the remaining cheese and mixture.
6. Serve warm.


**Nutrition:**

Calories:153 Net Carb:0.6g Fat:12.2g Saturated Fat: Carbohydrates: 0.7g Dietary Fiber: 0.1g Sugar: 0.4g Protein: 10.3g

# Chicken Chaffles

Preparation time: 10 minutes

Cooking Time: 15 Minutes

Servings: 2

## Ingredients:

- 2 oz chicken breasts, cooked, shredded
- 1/2 cup mozzarella cheese, finely shredded
- 2 eggs
- 6 tbsp parmesan cheese, finely shredded
- 1 cup zucchini, grated
- ½ cup almond flour
- 1tsp baking powder
- ¼ tsp garlic powder
- ¼ tsp black pepper, ground
- ½ tsp Italian seasoning
- ¼ tsp salt

## Directions:

1. Sprinkle the zucchini with a pinch of salt and set it aside for a few minutes. Squeeze out the excess water.
2. Warm up your mini waffle maker.
3. Mix chicken, almond flour, baking powder, cheeses, garlic powder, salt, pepper and seasonings in a bowl.
4. Use another small bow for beating eggs. Add them to squeezed zucchini, mix well.
5. Combine the chicken and egg mixture, and mix.
6. For a crispy crust, add a teaspoon of shredded cheese to the waffle maker and cook for 30 seconds.
7. Then, pour the mixture into the waffle maker and cook for 5 minutes or until crispy.
8. Carefully remove. Repeat with remaining batter the same steps.
9. Enjoy!

**Nutrition:**

Calories per Preparation time: 5 minutes35 Kcal ; Fats:g ; Carbs: 3 g ; Protein: 11 g

# Garlicky Chicken Chaffles

Preparation time: 6 minutes

Cooking Time: 12 Minutes

Servings: 2

## Ingredients:

- 1 organic egg, beaten
- 1/3 cup grass-fed cooked chicken, chopped
- 1/3 cup Mozzarella cheese, shredded
- ¼ teaspoon garlic, minced
- ¼ teaspoon dried basil, crushed

## Directions:

1. Preheat a mini waffle iron and then grease it.
2. In a bowl, place all the ingredients and mix until well combined.
3. Place half of the mixture into preheated waffle iron and cook for about 4-6 minutes or until golden brown.
4. Repeat with the remaining mixture.
5. Serve warm.

**Nutrition:**

Calories:81    Net    Carb:0.5g    Fat:3.7g    Saturated    Fat:1.4g
Carbohydrates: 0.5g Dietary Fiber: 0g Sugar: 0.2gProtein: 10.9g

# Garlic Herb Chaffles

Preparation time: 6 minutes

Cooking Time: 8 Minutes

Servings: 2

## Ingredients:

- 1 large organic egg, beaten
- ¼ cup Parmesan cheese, shredded
- ¼ cup Mozzarella cheese, shredded
- ½ tablespoon butter, melted
- 1 teaspoon garlic herb blend seasoning
- Salt, to taste

## Directions:

1. Preheat a mini waffle iron and then grease it.
2. In a bowl, place all the ingredients and beat until well combined.
3. Place half of the mixture into preheated waffle iron and cook for about 4 minutes or until golden brown.
4. Repeat with the remaining mixture.
5. Serve warm.

## Nutrition:

Calories:115   Net   Carb:1.1g   Fat:8.8g   Saturated   Fat:4.7g
Carbohydrates: 1.2g Dietary Fiber: 0.1g Sugar: 0.2g Protein: 8g

# Protein Cheddar Chaffles

Servings: 8

Cooking Time: 48 Minutes

**Ingredients:**

- ½ cup golden flax seeds meal
- ½ cup almond flour
- 2 tablespoons unflavored whey protein powder
- 1 teaspoon organic baking powder
- Salt and ground black pepper, to taste
- ¾ cup cheddar cheese, shredded
- 1/3 cup unsweetened almond milk
- 2 tablespoons unsalted butter, melted
- 2 large organic eggs, beaten

**Directions:**

1. Preheat a mini waffle iron and then grease it.
2. In a large bowl, add flax seeds meal, flour, protein powder, and baking powder, and mix well.
3. Stir in the cheddar cheese.

4. In another bowl, add the remaining ingredients and beat until well combined.
5. Add the egg mixture into the bowl with flax seeds meal mixture and mix until well combined.
6. Place desired amount of the mixture into preheated waffle iron.
7. Cook for about 4–6 minutes.
8. Repeat with the remaining mixture.
9. Serve warm.

## Nutrition:

Calories 187 Net Carbs 1.8 g Total Fat 14.5 g Saturated Fat 5 g Cholesterol 65 mg Sodium 134 mg Total Carbs 4.9 g Fiber 3.1 g Sugar 0.4 g Protein 8 g

# Garlic & Onion Powder Chaffles

Preparation time: 5 minutes

Cooking Time: 5 Minutes

Servings: 2

**Ingredients:**

- 1 organic egg, beaten
- ¼ cup Cheddar cheese, shredded
- 2 tablespoons almond flour
- ½ teaspoon organic baking powder
- ¼ teaspoon garlic powder
- ¼ teaspoon onion powder
- Pinch of salt

**Directions:**

1. Preheat a waffle iron and then grease it.
2. In a bowl, place all the ingredients and beat until well combined.
3. Place the mixture into preheated waffle iron and cook for about 5 minutes or until golden brown.

4. Serve warm.

## Nutrition:

Calories:274   Net   Carb:3.3g   Fat:21.3g   Saturated   Fat:7.8g
Carbohydrates: Dietary Fiber: 1.7g Sugar: 1.4g Protein: 12.8g

# Savory Bagel Seasoning Chaffles

Servings:4

Cooking Time: 5 Minutes

## Ingredients:

- 2 tbsps. everything bagel seasoning
- 2 eggs
- 1 cup mozzarella cheese
- 1/2 cup grated parmesan

## Directions:

1. Preheat the square waffle maker and grease with cooking spray.
2. Mix together eggs, mozzarella cheese and grated cheese in a bowl.
3. Pour half of the batter in the waffle maker.
4. Sprinkle 1 tbsp. of the everything bagel seasoning over batter.
5. Close the lid.
6. Cook chaffles for about 3-4 minutes Utes.

7. Repeat with the remaining batter.

8. Serve hot and enjoy!

**Nutrition:**

Protein: 34% 71 kcal Fat: 60% 125 kcal Carbohydrates: 6% 13 kcal

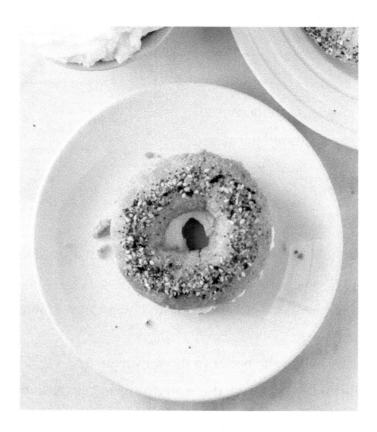

# Dried Herbs Chaffles

Preparation time: 6 minutes

Cooking Time: 8 Minutes

Servings: 2

## Ingredients:

- 1 organic egg, beaten
- ½ cup Cheddar cheese, shredded
- 1 tablespoon almond flour
- Pinch of dried thyme, crushed
- Pinch of dried rosemary, crushed

## Directions:

1. Preheat a mini waffle iron and then grease it.
2. In a bowl, place all the ingredients and beat until well combined.
3. Place half of the mixture into preheated waffle iron and cook for about 4 minutes or until golden brown.
4. Repeat with the remaining mixture.
5. Serve warm.

**Nutrition:**

Calories:1   Net   Carb:0.9g   Fat:13.4g   Saturated   Fat:6.8g
Carbohydrates: 1.3g Dietary Fiber: 0.4g Sugar: 0.4g Protein:
9.8g

# Sour Cream Protein Chaffles

Preparation time: 10 minutes

Cooking Time: 16 Minutes

Servings: 2

**Ingredients:**

- 6 organic eggs
- ½ cup sour cream
- ½ cup unsweetened whey protein powder
- 1 teaspoon organic baking powder
- ½ teaspoon salt
- 1 cup Cheddar cheese, shredded

**Directions:**

1. Preheat a waffle iron and then grease it.
2. In a medium bowl, place all ingredients and mix until well combined.
3. Place ¼ of the mixture into preheated waffle iron and cook for about 4 minutes or until golden brown.
4. Repeat with the remaining mixture.

5. Serve warm.


## Nutrition:

Calories:324 Net Carb:3. Fat:22.6g Saturated Fat:11.9g Carbohydrates: 3.6g Dietary Fiber: 0g Sugar: 1.3g Protein: 27.3g

# Zucchini & Basil Chaffles

Preparation time: 6 minutes

Cooking Time: 10 Minutes

Servings: 2

## Ingredients:

- 1 organic egg, beaten
- ¼ cup Mozzarella cheese, shredded
- 2 tablespoons Parmesan cheese, grated
- ½ of small zucchini, grated and squeezed
- ¼ teaspoon dried basil, crushed
- Freshly ground black pepper, as required

## Directions:

1. Preheat a mini waffle iron and then grease it.
2. In a medium bowl, place all ingredients and mix until well combined.
3. Place half of the mixture into preheated waffle iron and cook for about 4-5 minutes or until golden brown.
4. Repeat with the remaining mixture.

5. Serve warm.

## Nutrition:

Calories: Net Carb: 1g Fat: 4.1g Saturated Fat: 1.7g Carbohydrates: 1.3g Dietary Fiber: 0.3g Sugar: 0.7g Protein: 6.1g

# Hash Brown Chaffle

Preparation time: 6 minutes

Cooking Time: 10 Minutes

Servings: 2

## Ingredients:

- 1 large jicama root, peeled and shredded
- ½ medium onion, minced
- 2 garlic cloves, pressed
- 1 cup cheddar shredded cheese
- 2 eggs
- Salt and pepper, to taste

## Directions:

1. Place jicama in a colander, sprinkle with 2 tsp salt, and let drain.
2. Squeeze out all excess liquid.
3. Microwave jicama for 5-8 minutes.
4. Mix ¾ of cheese and all other ingredients in a bowl.

5. Sprinkle 1-2 tsp cheese on waffle maker, add 3 Tbsp mixture, and top with 1-2 tsp cheese.
6. Cook for 5-minutes, or until done.
7. Remove and repeat for remaining batter.
8. Serve while hot with preferred toppings.

**Nutrition:**

Carbs: g ; Fat: 6 g ; Protein: 4 g ; Calories: 194

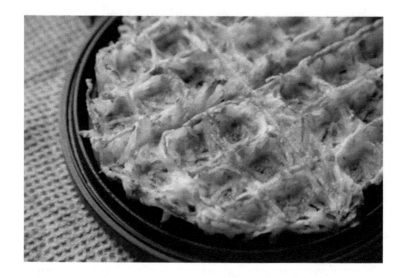

# Grilled Cheese Chaffle

Preparation time: 3 minutes

Cooking time: 8 minutes

Servings: 1

## Ingredients:

- 1 egg
- 1/4 teaspoon garlic powder
- 1/2 cup shred cheddar
- 2 American cheese or 1/4 cup shredded cheese
- 1 tablespoon butter

## Directions

1. In a small bowl, mix bacon, garlic powder and shredded cheddar cheese.
2. After heating the dash waffle maker, add half the mixture of the scramble. Cook and cook for 4 minutes.
3. Add to the dash mini waffle maker the remainder of the scramble mixture and cook for 4 minutes.

4. Steam the stove pan over moderate heat when both chaffles are finished.

5. Attach 1 spoonful of butter and dissolve. Place one chaffle in the pan once the butter has melted. Place your favorite cheese on top of the chaffle and finish with a second chaffle.

6. Cook the chaffle for 1 minute on the first side, turn it over and cook for another 1-2 minutes on the other side to finish the cheese melting.

7. Cut it from the bread when the cheese melts and eat it!

## Nutrition:

Calories: 549kcal carbohydrates: 3g protein: 27g fats: 48gsaturated fats: 28g cholesterol: 295mg sodium: 1216mg potassium: 172mg sugar: 1g

# Baked Potato Chaffle Using Jicama

Preparation time: 20 minutes

Cooking time: 7 minutes

Servings: 1

## Ingredients:

- 1 jicama root
- 1/2 onion, medium, minced
- 2 cloves garlic, pressed
- 1 cup cheese
- 1 eggs, whisked
- Salt and pepper

## Directions:

1. Peel the jicama root and shred it using a food processor.
2. Place the shredded jicama root in a colander to allow the water to drain. Mix in 2 tsp of salt as well.
3. Squeeze out the remaining liquid.

4. Microwave the shredded jicama for 5-8 minutes. This step pre-cooks it.

5. Mix all the remaining Ingredients together with the jicama.

6. Start preheating the waffle maker.

7. Once preheated, sprinkle a bit of cheese on the waffle maker, allowing it to toast for a few seconds.

8. Place 3 tbsp of the jicama mixture onto the waffle maker. Sprinkle more cheese on top before closing the lid.

9. Cook for 5 minutes. Flip the chaffle and let it cook for 2 more minutes.

10. Servings your baked jicama by topping it with sour cream, cheese, bacon pieces, and chives.

## Nutrition:

calories: 168 carbohydrates: 5.1g fat: 11.8g protein: 10g

# Tiramisu Chaffle

Preparation time: 6 hrs

Cooking time: 6 mins

Servings: 8

## Ingredients:

- 2 eggs
- 2 oz cream cheese, softened
- 1 tbsp coconut flour
- 1 tbsp heavy cream
- 1 tsp vanilla extract
- 1/2 tsp baking powder
- 1/2 tsp ground cinnamon
- 1/4 tsp stevia powder

## For the coffee syrup:

- 4 tbsp strong coffee
- 5 drops liquid stevia

## For the filling:

- 1 oz cream cheese, softened
- 3 oz mascarpone cheese, softened

- 1/4 cup heavy cream
- 2 tsp vanilla extract
- 1/4 tsp stevia powder

**For dusting:**

- 1/2 tsp unsweetened cocoa powder

**Directions:**

1. Preheat the mini waffle maker.
2. Combine all the chaffle Ingredients in a blender.
3. Once the waffle maker is heated, pour about 1/4 of the batter and allow it to cook for 5-6 minutes. Remove the cooked chaffle and repeat this step for the remaining batter.
4. While waiting for the chaffle to cook, mix the liquid stevia and coffee in a small bowl for the coffee syrup.
5. For the filling, mix the vanilla, stevia powder, and heavy cream. Whisk this until soft peaks start to form.
6. In a separate mixing bowl, use a hand mixer to combine the mascarpone and cream cheese. Once done, mix it in with the whipped cream.
7. To assemble, drizzle 1 tbsp of coffee syrup on the chaffle.

8. On one chaffle, spread a quarter of the filling. Top this with another chaffle, and repeat the previous step until you have four layers of chaffles.

9. Dust the finished tiramisu chaffle with the unsweetened cocoa powder.

10. Refrigerate this for 6 hours or more before serving.

## Nutrition:

calories: 567 carbohydrate: 6.6g fat: 53.4g protein: 14.7g

# Spicy Jalapeno Popper Chaffles

Preparation time: 10 mins

Cooking time: 10 mins

Servings: 1

## Ingredients: for the chaffles:

- 1 egg
- 1 oz cream cheese, softened
- 1 cup cheddar cheese, shredded

## For the toppings:

- 2 tbsp bacon bits
- 1/2 tbsp jalapenos

## Directions:

1. Turn on the waffle maker. Preheat for up to 5 minutes.
2. Mix the chaffle Ingredients.
3. Pour the batter onto the waffle maker.
4. Cook the batter for 3-4 minutes until it's brown and crispy.

5. Remove the chaffle and repeat steps until all remaining batter have been used up.

6. Sprinkle bacon bits and a few jalapeno slices as toppings.

## Nutrition:

calories: 231 carbohydrate: 2g fat: 18g protein: 13g

# Eggnog Chaffles

Preparation time: 15 minutes

Cooking time: 10 minutes

Servings: 1

## Ingredients:

- 1 egg, separated
- 1 egg yolk
- 1/2 cup mozzarella cheese Shredded
- 1/2 tsp spiced rum
- 1 tsp vanilla extract
- 1/4 tsp nutmeg, dried
- A dash of cinnamon
- 1 tsp coconut flour

## For the icing:

- 2 tbsp cream cheese
- 1 tbsp powdered sweetener
- 2 tsp rum or rum extract

## Directions:

1. Preheat the mini waffle maker.
2. Mix egg yolk in a small bowl until smooth.
3. Add in the sweetener and mix until the powder is completely dissolved.
4. Add the coconut flour, cinnamon, and nutmeg. Mix well.In another bowl, mix rum, egg white, and vanilla. Whisk until well combined.
5. Throw in the yolk mixture with the egg white mixture. You should be able to form a thin batter.
6. Add the mozzarella cheese and combine with the mixture.
7. Separate the batter into two batches. Put 1/2 of the batter into the waffle maker and let it cook for 6 minutes until it's solid.
8. Repeat until you've used up the remaining batter.
9. In a separate bowl, mix all the icing Ingredients.
10. Top the cooked chaffles with the icing, or you can use this as a dip.

## Nutrition:

calories: 266 carbohydrates: 2g fat: 23g protein: 13g

# Cheddar Jalapeno Chaffles

Preparation time: 15 minutes

Cooking time: 10 minutes

Servings: 1

## Ingredients:

- 1 egg
- 1/2 cup cheddar cheese shredded
- 1 tbsp almond flour
- 1 tbsp jalapenos
- 1 tbsp olive oil

## Directions:

1. Preheat the waffle maker.
2. While waiting for the waffle maker to heat up, mix jalapeno, egg, cheese, and almond flour in a small mixing bowl.
3. Lightly grease the waffle maker with olive oil.
4. In the center of the waffle maker, carefully pour the chaffle batter. Spread the mixture evenly toward the edges.

5. Close the waffle maker lid and wait for 3-4 minutes for the mixture to cook. For an even crispier texture, wait for another 1-2 minutes.

6. Remove the chaffle. Let it cool before serving.

**Nutrition:**

calories: 509 carbohydrates: 5g fat: 45g protein: 23g

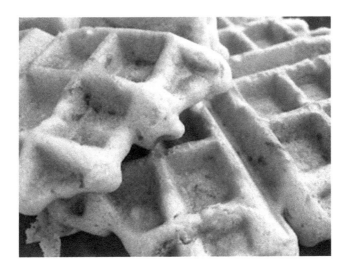

# Low Carb Keto Broccoli Cheese Waffles

Preparation time: 5 minutes

Cooking time: 5 minutes

Servings: 2

## Ingredients:

- 1 cup broccoli, processed
- 1 cup shredded cheddar cheese
- 1/3 cup grated parmesan cheese
- 2 eggs, beats

## Directions

1. Spray the Cooking spray on the waffle iron and preheat.
2. Use a powerful blender or food processor to process the broccoli until rice consistency.
3. Mix all Ingredients in a medium bowl.
4. Add 1/3 of the mixture to the waffle iron and cook for 4-5 minutes until golden.

## Nutrition:

Calories 160 Total fat 11.8g 18% Cholesterol 121mg 40% Sodium 221.8mg 9% Total carbohydrate 5.1g 2% Dietary fiber 1.7g 7% Sugars 1.2g Protein 10g 20% Vitamin a 133.5µg 9% Vitamin c 7.3mg 12%

# Strawberry Cream Sandwich Chaffles

Preparation time: 6 minutes

Servings: 2

Cooking Time: 6 Minutes

## Ingredients:

### Chaffles

- 1 large organic egg, beaten
- ½ cup mozzarella cheese, shredded finely Filling
- 4 teaspoons heavy cream
- 2 tablespoons powdered erythritol
- 1 teaspoon fresh lemon juice
- Pinch of fresh lemon zest, grated
- 2 fresh strawberries, hulled and sliced

## Directions:

1. Preheat a mini waffle iron and then grease it.

2. For chaffles: in a small bowl, add the egg and mozzarella cheese and stir to combine.

3. Place half of the mixture into preheated waffle iron and cook for about 2–minutes.

4. Repeat with the remaining mixture.

5. Meanwhile, for filling: in a bowl, place all the ingredients except the strawberry slices and with a hand mixer, beat until well combined.

6. Serve each chaffle with cream mixture and strawberry slices.

## Nutrition:

Calories 95 Net Carbs 1.4 g Total Fat 5 g Saturated Fat 3.9 g Cholesterol 110 mg Sodium 82 mg Total Carbs 1.7 g Fiber 0.3 g Sugar 0.9 g Protein 5.5 g

# Ham Sandwich Chaffles

Preparation time: 6 minutes

Servings: 2

Cooking Time: 8 Minutes

## Ingredients:

- 1 organic egg, beaten
- ½ cup Monterrey Jack cheese, shredded
- 1 teaspoon coconut flour
- Pinch of garlic powder

## Filling

- 2 sugar-free ham slices
- 1 small tomato, sliced
- 2 lettuce leaves

## Directions:

1. Preheat a mini waffle iron and then grease it.
2. For chaffles: In a medium bowl, put all ingredients and with a fork, mix until well combined. Place half of the

mixture into preheated waffle iron and cook for about 3–4 minutes.

3. Repeat with the remaining mixture.

4. Serve each chaffle with filling ingredients.


**Nutrition:**

Calories 1 Net Carbs 3.7 g Total Fat 8.7 g Saturated Fat 3.4 g Cholesterol 114 mg Sodium 794 mg Total Carbs 5.5 g Fiber 1.8 g Sugar 1.5 g Protein 13.9 g

# Chicken Sandwich Chaffles

Preparation time: 6 minutes.

Servings: 2

Cooking Time: 8 Minutes

**Ingredients:**

**Chaffles**

- 1 large organic egg, beaten
- ½ cup cheddar cheese, shredded
- Pinch of salt and ground black pepper

**Filling**

- 1 (6-ounce) cooked chicken breast, halved
- 2 lettuce leaves
- ¼ of small onion, sliced
- 1 small tomato, sliced

**Directions:**

1. Preheat a mini waffle iron and then grease it.

2.  For chaffles: In a medium bowl, put all ingredients and with a fork, mix until well combined. Place half of the mixture into preheated waffle iron and cook for about 3–4 minutes.
3.  Repeat with the remaining mixture.
4.  Serve each chaffle with filling ingredients.

## Nutrition:

Calories 2 Net Carbs 2.5 g Total Fat 14.1 g Saturated Fat 6.8 g Cholesterol 177 mg Sodium 334 mg Total Carbs 3.3 g Fiber 0.8 g Sugar 2 g Protein 28.7 g

# Salmon & Cheese Sandwich Chaffles

Preparation time: 6 minutes

Servings: 4

Cooking Time: 24 Minutes

## Ingredients:

### Chaffles

- 2 organic eggs
- ½ ounce butter, melted
- 1 cup mozzarella cheese, shredded
- 2 tablespoons almond flour
- Pinch of salt

### Filling

- ½ cup smoked salmon
- 1/3 cup avocado, peeled, pitted, and sliced
- 2 tablespoons feta cheese, crumbled

## Directions:

1. Preheat a mini waffle iron and then grease it.
2. For chaffles: In a medium bowl, put all ingredients and with a fork, mix until well combined. Place ¼ of the mixture into preheated waffle iron and cook for about 5–6 minutes.
3. Repeat with the remaining mixture.
4. Serve each chaffle with filling ingredients.

## Nutrition:

Calories 169 Net Carbs 1.2 g Total Fat 13.g Saturated Fat 5 g Cholesterol 101 mg Sodium 319 mg Total Carbs 2.8 g Fiber 1.6 g Sugar 0.6 g Protein 8.9 g

# Strawberry Cream Cheese Sandwich Chaffles

Preparation time: 6 minutes

Servings: 2

Cooking Time: 10 Minutes

## Ingredients:

### Chaffles

- 1 organic egg, beaten
- 1 teaspoon organic vanilla extract
- 1 tablespoon almond flour
- 1 teaspoon organic baking powder
- Pinch of ground cinnamon
- 1 cup mozzarella cheese, shredded

### Filling

- 2 tablespoons cream cheese, softened
- 2 tablespoons erythritol
- ¼ teaspoon organic vanilla extract
- 2 fresh strawberries, hulled and chopped

## Directions:

1. Preheat a mini waffle iron and then grease it.
2. For chaffles: in a bowl, add the egg and vanilla extract and mix well.
3. Add the flour, baking powder, and cinnamon, and mix until well combined.
4. Add the mozzarella cheese and stir to combine.
5. Place half of the mixture into preheated waffle iron and cook for about 4–minutes.
6. Repeat with the remaining mixture.
7. Meanwhile, for filling: in a bowl, place all the ingredients except the strawberry pieces and with a hand mixer, beat until well combined.
8. Serve each chaffle with cream cheese mixture and strawberry pieces.

## Nutrition:

Calories 143 Net Carb: g Total Fat 10.1 g Saturated Fat 4.5 g Cholesterol 100 mg Sodium 148 mg Total Carbs 4.1 g Fiber 0.8 g Sugar 1.2 g Protein 7.6 g

# Egg & Bacon Sandwich Chaffles

Preparation time: 6 minutes

Servings: 4

Cooking Time: 20 Minutes

## Ingredients:

### Chaffles

- 2 large organic eggs, beaten
- 4 tablespoons almond flour
- 1 teaspoon organic baking powder
- 1 cup mozzarella cheese, shredded

### Filling

- 4 organic fried eggs
- 4 cooked bacon slices

## Directions:

1. Preheat a mini waffle iron and then grease it.

2. In a medium bowl, put all ingredients and with a fork, mix until well combined. Place half of the mixture into preheated waffle iron and cook for about 3–5 minutes.
3. Repeat with the remaining mixture.
4. Repeat with the remaining mixture.
5. Serve each chaffle with filling ingredients.


**Nutrition:**

Calories 197 Net Carb: g Total Fat 14.5 g Saturated Fat 4.1 g Cholesterol 2 mg Sodium 224 g Total Carbs 2.7 g Fiber 0.8 g Sugar 0.8 g Protein 12.9 g

# Blueberry Peanut Butter Sandwich Chaffles

Preparation time: 6 minutes

Servings: 2

Cooking Time: 10 Minutes

### Ingredients:

- 1 organic egg, beaten
- ½ cup cheddar cheese, shredded

### Filling

- 2 tablespoons erythritol
- 1 tablespoon butter, softened
- 1 tablespoon natural peanut butter
- 2 tablespoons cream cheese, softened
- ¼ teaspoon organic vanilla extract
- 2 teaspoons fresh blueberries

## Directions:

1. Preheat a mini waffle iron and then grease it.

## For chaffles:

2. in a small bowl, add the egg and Cheddar cheese and stir to combine.
3. Place half of the mixture into preheated waffle iron and cook for about 5 minutes.
4. Repeat with the remaining mixture.
5. Meanwhile, for filling: In a medium bowl, put all ingredients and mix until well combined.
6. Serve each chaffle with peanut butter mixture.

## Nutrition:

Calories 143 Net Carbs 3.3 g Total Fat 10.1 g Saturated Fat 4.5 g Cholesterol 100 mg Sodium 148 mg Total Carbs 4.1 g Fiber 0.8 g Sugar 1.2 g Protein 6 g

# Chocolate Sandwich Chaffles

Preparation time: 6 minutes

Servings: 2

Cooking Time: 10 Minutes

**Ingredients:**

**Chaffles**

- 1 organic egg, beaten
- 1 ounce cream cheese, softened
- 2 tablespoons almond flour
- 1 tablespoon cacao powder
- 2 teaspoons erythritol
- 1 teaspoon organic vanilla extract

**Filling**

- 2 tablespoons cream cheese, softened
- 2 tablespoons erythritol
- ½ tablespoon cacao powder
- ¼ teaspoon organic vanilla extract

## Directions:

1. Preheat a mini waffle iron and then grease it.

## For chaffles:

2. In a medium bowl, put all ingredients and with a fork, mix until well combined. Place half of the mixture into preheated waffle iron and cook for about 3–5 minutes.
3. Repeat with the remaining mixture.
4. Meanwhile, for filling: In a medium bowl, put all ingredients and with a hand mixer, beat until well combined.
5. Serve each chaffle with chocolate mixture.

## Nutrition:

Calories 192 Net Carb: g Total Fat 16 g Saturated Fat 7.6 g Cholesterol 113 mg Sodium 115 mg Total Carbs 4.4 g Fiber 1.9 g Sugar 0.8 g Protein 5.7 g

# Berry Sauce Sandwich Chaffles

Preparation time: 6 minutes

Servings: 2

Cooking Time: 8 Minutes

## Ingredients:

### Filling

- 3 ounces frozen mixed berries, thawed with the juice
- 1 tablespoon erythritol
- 1 tablespoon water
- ¼ tablespoon fresh lemon juice
- 2 teaspoons cream

### Chaffles

- 1 large organic egg, beaten
- ½ cup cheddar cheese, shredded
- 2 tablespoons almond flour

## Directions:

### For berry sauce:

1. In a pan, add the berries, erythritol, water and lemon juice over medium heat and cook for about 8– minutes, pressing with the spoon occasionally.
2. Remove the pan of sauce from heat and set aside to cool before serving.
3. Preheat a mini waffle iron and then grease it.
4. In a bowl, add the egg, cheddar cheese and almond flour and beat until well combined. Place half of the mixture into preheated waffle iron and cook for about 3–5 minutes.
5. Repeat with the remaining mixture.
6. Serve each chaffle with cream and berry sauce.

## Nutrition:

Calories 222 Net Carbs 4.g Total Fat 16 g Saturated Fat 7.2 g Cholesterol 123 mg Sodium 212 mg Total Carbs 7 g Fiber 2.3 g Sugar 3.8 g Protein 10.5 g

# Pork Sandwich Chaffles

Preparation time: 6 minutes

Servings: 4

Cooking Time: 16 Minutes

## Ingredients:

### Chaffles

- 2 large organic eggs
- ¼ cup superfine blanched almond flour
- ¾ teaspoon organic baking powder
- ½ teaspoon garlic powder
- 1 cup cheddar cheese, shredded

### Filling

- 12 ounces cooked pork, cut into slices
- 1 tomato, sliced
- 4 lettuce leaves

## Directions:

1. Preheat a mini waffle iron and then grease it.

## For chaffles:

2. In a bowl, add the eggs, almond flour, baking powder, and garlic powder, and beat until well combined.
3. Add the cheese and stir to combine.
4. Place ¼ of the mixture into preheated waffle iron and cook for about 3–minutes.
5. Repeat with the remaining mixture.
6. Serve each chaffle with filling ingredients.

## Nutrition:

Calories 319 Net Carbs 2.5 g Total Fat 18.2 g Saturated Fat 8 g Cholesterol 185 mg Sodium 263 mg Total Carbs 3.5 g Fiber 1 g Sugar 0.9 g Protein 34.2 g

# Tomato Sandwich Chaffles

Preparation time: 6 minutes

Servings: 2

Cooking Time: 6 Minutes

**Ingredients:**

**Chaffles**

- 1 large organic egg, beaten
- ½ cup colby jack cheese, shredded finely
- 1/8 teaspoon organic vanilla extract

**Filling**

- 1 small tomato, sliced
- 2 teaspoons fresh basil leaves

**Directions:**

1. Preheat a mini waffle iron and then grease it.

**For chaffles:**

2. in a small bowl, place all the ingredients and stir to combine.
3. Place half of the mixture into preheated waffle iron and cook for about minutes.
4. Repeat with the remaining mixture.
5. Serve each chaffle with tomato slices and basil leaves.

**Nutrition:**

Calories 155 Net Carbs 2.4 g Total Fat 11.g Saturated Fat 6.8 g Cholesterol 118 mg Sodium 217 mg Total Carbs 3 g Fiber 0.6 g Sugar 1.4 g Protein 9.6 g

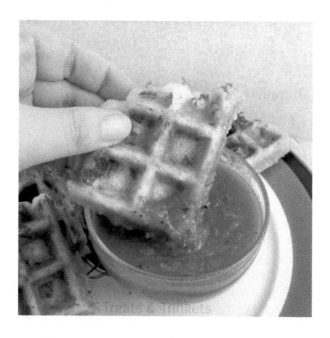

# Chocolate Chaffle Cake

Preparation time: 6 minutes

Servings: 2

Cooking Time: 8 Minutes

**Ingredients:**

**Chocolate Chaffle Cake Ingredients:**

- 2 tablespoons cocoa powder
- 2 tablespoons Swerve granulated sweetener
- 1 egg
- 1 tablespoon heavy whipping cream
- 1 tablespoon almond flour
- 1/4 tsp baking powder
- 1/2 tsp vanilla extract

**Cream Cheese Frosting:**

- 2 tablespoons cream cheese
- 2 teaspoons swerve confectioners
- 1/8 tsp vanilla extract
- 1 tsp heavy cream

**Directions:**

**How to Make Chocolate Chaffle Cake:**

1. In a small bowl, whisk together cocoa powder, swerve, almond flour, and baking powder.
2. Add in the vanilla extract and heavy whipping cream and mix well.
3. Add in the egg and mix well. Be sure to scrape the sides of the bowl to get all of the ingredients mixed well.
4. Let sit for 3-4 minutes while the mini waffle maker heats up.
5. Add half of the waffle mixture to the waffle maker and cook for 4 minutes. Then cook the second waffle. While the second chocolate keto waffle is cooking, make your frosting.

**How to Make Cream Cheese Frosting:**

6. In a small microwave-safe bowl add 2 tablespoons cream cheese. Microwave the cream cheese for seconds to soften the cream cheese.
7. Add in heavy whipping cream and vanilla extract and use a small hand mixer to mix well.
8. Then add in the confectioners swerve and use the hand mixer to incorporate and fluffy the frosting.

**Assembling Keto Chocolate Chaffle cake:**

9. Place one chocolate chaffle on a plate, top with a layer of frosting. You can spread it with a knife or use a pastry bag and pipe the frosting.

10. Put the second chocolate chaffle on top of the frosting layer and then spread or pipe the rest of the frosting on top.

**Nutrition:**

(perserving): Calories:   151kcal; Carbohydrates:5g; Protein:6g; Fat: 13g ; Saturated Fat:6g ; Cholesterol:111mg ; Sodium:83mg ; Potassium:190mg  ; Fiber: 2g  ; Sugar: 1g  ; Vitamin A: 461IU ; Calcium: 67mg  ; Iron:1mg

# Salmon & Cream Sandwich Chaffles

Preparation time: 6 minutes

Servings: 2

Cooking Time: 8 Minutes

## Ingredients:

### Chaffles

- 1 organic egg, beaten
- ½ cup cheddar cheese, shredded
- 1 tablespoon almond flour
- 1 tablespoon fresh rosemary, chopped

### Filling

- ¼ cup smoked salmon
- 1 teaspoon fresh dill, chopped
- 2 tablespoons cream

## Directions:

1. Preheat a mini waffle iron and then grease it.
2. For chaffles: In a medium bowl, put all ingredients and with a fork, mix until well combined. Place half of the mixture into preheated waffle iron and cook for about 3–4 minutes.
3. Repeat with the remaining mixture.
4. Serve each chaffle with filling ingredients.

## Nutrition:

Calories 202 Net Carbs 1.7 g Total Fat 11 g Saturated Fat 7.5 g Cholesterol 118 mg Sodium 345 mg Total Carbs 2.9 g Fiber 1.2 g Sugar 0.7 g Protein 13.2 g

# Tuna Sandwich Chaffles

Preparation time: 6 minutes

Servings: 2

Cooking Time: 8 Minutes

## Ingredients:

### Chaffles

- 1 organic egg, beaten
- ½ cup cheddar cheese, shredded
- 1 tablespoon almond flour
- Pinch of salt

### Filling

- ¼ cup water-packed tuna, flaked
- 2 lettuce leaves

## Directions:

1. Preheat a mini waffle iron and then grease it.
2. For chaffles: In a medium bowl, put all ingredients and with a fork, mix until well combined. Place half of the

mixture into preheated waffle iron and cook for about 3–4 minutes.

3. Repeat with the remaining mixture.
4. Serve each chaffle with filling ingredients.


## Nutrition:

Calories 186 Net Carbs 0.9 g Total Fat 13.6 g Saturated Fat 6.8 g Cholesterol 120 mg Sodium 342 mg Total Carbs 1.3 g Fiber 0.4 g Sugar 0.g Protein 13.6 g

# Pork Chops on Chaffle

Preparation time: 10 minutes

Cooking Time:15 Minutes

Servings: 2

**Ingredients:**

- 4 eggs
- 2 cups grated mozzarella cheese
- Salt and pepper to taste
- Pinch of nutmeg
- 2 tablespoons sour cream
- 6 tablespoons almond flour
- 2 teaspoons baking powder
- Pork chops
- 2 tablespoons olive oil
- 1 pound pork chops
- Salt and pepper to taste
- 1 teaspoon freshly chopped rosemary

## Other

- 2 tablespoons cooking spray to brush the waffle maker
- 2 tablespoons freshly chopped basil for decoration

## Directions:

1. Preheat the waffle maker.
2. Add the eggs, mozzarella cheese, salt and pepper, nutmeg, sour cream, almond flour and baking powder to a bowl.
3. Mix until combined.
4. Brush the heated waffle maker with cooking spray and add a few tablespoons of the batter.
5. Close the lid and cook for about 7 minutes depending on your waffle maker.
6. Meanwhile, heat the butter in a nonstick grill pan and season the pork chops with salt and pepper and freshly chopped rosemary.
7. Cook the pork chops for about 4–5 minutes on each side.
8. Serve each chaffle with a pork chop and sprinkle some freshly chopped basil on top.

**Nutrition**: Calories 666, fat 55.2 g, carbs 4.8 g, sugar 0.4 g, Protein 37.5 g, sodium 235 mg

# Classic Beef Chaffle

Preparation time: 10 minutes

Cooking Time:10 Minutes

Servings: 2

**Ingredients:**

**Batter**

- ½ pound ground beef
- 4 eggs
- 4 ounces cream cheese
- 1 cup grated mozzarella cheese
- Salt and pepper to taste
- 1 clove garlic, minced
- ½ teaspoon freshly chopped rosemary

**Other**

- 2 tablespoons butter to brush the waffle maker
- ¼ cup sour cream
- 2 tablespoons freshly chopped parsley for garnish

## Directions:

1. Preheat the waffle maker.
2. Add the ground beef, eggs, cream cheese, grated mozzarella cheese, salt and pepper, minced garlic and freshly chopped rosemary to a bowl.
3. Brush the heated waffle maker with butter and add a few tablespoons of the batter.
4. Close the lid and cook for about 8–10 minutes depending on your waffle maker.
5. Serve each chaffle with a tablespoon of sour cream and freshly chopped parsley on top.
6. Serve and enjoy.

## Nutrition:

Calories 368, fat 24 g, carbs 2.1 g, sugar 0.4 g, Protein 27.4 g, sodium 291 mg

# Beef and Tomato Chaffle

Preparation time: 10 minutes

Cooking Time:15 Minutes

Servings: 2

## Ingredients:

### Batter

- 4 eggs
- ¼ cup cream cheese
- 1 cup grated mozzarella cheese
- Salt and pepper to taste
- ¼ cup almond flour
- 1 teaspoon freshly chopped dill
- Beef
- 1 pound beef loin
- Salt and pepper to taste
- 1 tablespoon balsamic vinegar
- 2 tablespoons olive oil
- 1 teaspoon freshly chopped rosemary

## Other

- 2 tablespoons cooking spray to brush the waffle maker
- 4 tomato slices for serving

## Directions:

1. Preheat the waffle maker.
2. Add the eggs, cream cheese, grated mozzarella cheese, salt and pepper, almond flour and freshly chopped dill to a bowl.
3. Mix until combined and batter forms.
4. Brush the heated waffle maker with cooking spray and add a few tablespoons of the batter.
5. Close the lid and cook for about 8–10 minutes depending on your waffle maker.
6. Meanwhile, heat the olive oil in a nonstick frying pan and season the beef loin with salt and pepper and freshly chopped rosemary.
7. Cook the beef on each side for about 5 minutes and drizzle with some balsamic vinegar.
8. Serve each chaffle with a slice of tomato and cooked beef loin slices.

**Nutrition:** Calories 4, fat 35.8 g, carbs 3.3 g, sugar 0.8 g, Protein 40.3 g, sodium 200 mg

# Classic Ground Pork Chaffle

Preparation time: 10 minutes

Cooking Time:15 Minutes

Servings: 2

## Ingredients:

- ½ pound ground pork
- 3 eggs
- ½ cup grated mozzarella cheese
- Salt and pepper to taste
- 1 clove garlic, minced
- 1 teaspoon dried oregano
- Other
- 2 tablespoons butter to brush the waffle maker
- 2 tablespoons freshly chopped parsley for garnish

## Directions:

1. Preheat the waffle maker.
2. Add the ground pork, eggs, mozzarella cheese, salt and pepper, minced garlic and dried oregano to a bowl.

3. Mix until combined.

4. Brush the heated waffle maker with butter and add a few tablespoons of the batter.

5. Close the lid and cook for about 7–8 minutes depending on your waffle maker.

6. Serve with freshly chopped parsley.

**Nutrition:**

Calories 192, fat 11.g, carbs 1 g, sugar 0.3 g, Protein 20.2 g, sodium 142 mg

# Ground Chicken Chaffle

Preparation time: 10 minutes

Cooking Time:8–10 Minutes

Servings: 2

## Ingredients:

### Batter

- ½ pound ground chicken
- 4 eggs
- 3 tablespoons tomato sauce
- Salt and pepper to taste
- 1 cup grated mozzarella cheese
- 1 teaspoon dried oregano

### Other

- 2 tablespoons butter to brush the waffle maker

## Directions:

1. Preheat the waffle maker.

2. Add the ground chicken, eggs and tomato sauce to a bowl and season with salt and pepper.
3. Mix everything with a fork and stir in the mozzarella cheese and dried oregano.
4. Mix again until fully combined.
5. Brush the heated waffle maker with butter and add a few tablespoons of the batter.
6. Close the lid and cook for about 8–10 minutes depending on your waffle maker.
7. Serve and enjoy.

**Nutrition:**

Calories 246, fat 15.6 g, carbs 1.5 g, sugar 0.9 g, Protein 24.2 g,

sodium 254 mg

# Beef Chaffle Taco

Preparation time: 10 minutes

Cooking Time:15 Minutes

Servings: 2

**Ingredients:**

**Batter**

- 4 eggs
- 2 cups grated cheddar cheese
- ¼ cup heavy cream
- Salt and pepper to taste
- ¼ cup almond flour
- 2 teaspoons baking powder
- Beef
- 2 tablespoons butter
- ½ onion, diced
- 1 pound ground beef
- Salt and pepper to taste
- 1 teaspoon dried oregano
- 1 tablespoon sugar-free ketchup

**Other**

- 2 tablespoons cooking spray to brush the waffle maker
- 2 tablespoons freshly chopped parsley

## Directions:

1. Preheat the waffle maker.
2. Add the eggs, grated cheddar cheese, heavy cream, salt and pepper, almond flour and baking powder to a bowl.
3. Brush the heated waffle maker with cooking spray and add a few tablespoons of the batter.
4. Close the lid and cook for about 5–7 minutes depending on your waffle maker.
5. Once the chaffle is ready, place it in a napkin holder to harden into the shape of a taco as it cools.
6. Meanwhile, melt and heat the butter in a nonstick frying pan and start cooking the diced onion.
7. Once the onion is tender, add the ground beef. Season with salt and pepper and dried oregano and stir in the sugar-free ketchup.
8. Cook for about 7 minutes.
9. Serve the cooked ground meat in each taco chaffle sprinkled with some freshly chopped parsley.

## Nutrition:

Calories 719, fat 51.7 g, carbs 7.3 g, sugar 1.3 g, Protein 56.1 g, sodium 573 mg

# Turkey Chaffle Sandwich

Preparation time: 10 minutes

Cooking Time:15 Minutes

Servings: 2

## Ingredients:

### Batter

- 4 eggs
- ¼ cup cream cheese
- 1 cup grated mozzarella cheese
- Salt and pepper to taste
- 1 teaspoon dried dill
- ½ teaspoon onion powder
- ½ teaspoon garlic powder
- Juicy chicken
- 2 tablespoons butter
- 1 pound chicken breast
- Salt and pepper to taste
- 1 teaspoon dried dill
- 2 tablespoons heavy cream

## Other

- 2 tablespoons butter to brush the waffle maker
- 4 lettuce leaves to garnish the sandwich
- 4 tomato slices to garnish the sandwich

## Directions:

1. Preheat the waffle maker.
2. Add the eggs, cream cheese, mozzarella cheese, salt and pepper, dried dill, onion powder and garlic powder to a bowl.
3. Mix everything with a fork just until batter forms.
4. Brush the heated waffle maker with butter and add a few tablespoons of the batter.
5. Close the lid and cook for about 7 minutes depending on your waffle maker.
6. Meanwhile, heat some butter in a nonstick pan.
7. Season the chicken with salt and pepper and sprinkle with dried dill. Pour the heavy cream on top.
8. Cook the chicken slices for about 10 minutes or until golden brown.
9. Cut each chaffle in half.
10. On one half add a lettuce leaf, tomato slice, and chicken slice. Cover with the other chaffle half to make a sandwich.

11. Serve and enjoy.

## Nutrition:

Calories 381, fat 26.3 g, carbs 2.5 g, sugar 1 g, Protein 32.9 g, sodium 278 mg

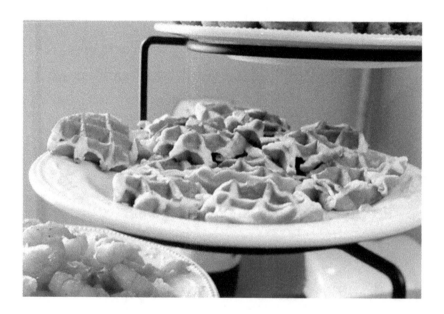

# Bbq Sauce Pork Chaffle

Preparation time: 10 minutes

Cooking Time:15 Minutes

Servings: 2

## Ingredients:

- ½ pound ground por
- 3 eggs
- 1 cup grated mozzarella cheese
- Salt and pepper to taste
- 1 clove garlic, minced
- 1 teaspoon dried rosemary
- 3 tablespoons sugar-free BBQ sauce

## Other

- 2 tablespoons butter to brush the waffle maker
- ½ pound pork rinds for serving
- ¼ cup sugar-free BBQ sauce for serving

## Directions:

1. Preheat the waffle maker.
2. Add the ground pork, eggs, mozzarella, salt and pepper, minced garlic, dried rosemary, and BBQ sauce to a bowl.
3. Mix until combined.
4. Brush the heated waffle maker with butter and add a few tablespoons of the batter.
5. Close the lid and cook for about 7–8 minutes depending on your waffle maker.
6. Serve each chaffle with some pork rinds and a tablespoon of BBQ sauce.

## Nutrition:

Calories 350, fat 21.1 g, carbs 2.g, sugar 0.3 g, Protein 36.9 g, sodium 801 mg

# Garlic Chicken Chaffle

Preparation time: 10 minutes

Cooking Time:15 Minutes

Servings: 2

## Ingredients:

### Batter

- 4 eggs
- 2 cups grated mozzarella cheese
- ¼ cup almond flour
- 2 tablespoons coconut flour
- 2½ teaspoons baking powder
- Salt and pepper to taste

### Garlic Chicken Topping

- 1 pound diced chicken
- Salt and pepper to taste
- 1 teaspoon dried oregano
- 2 garlic cloves, minced
- 3 tablespoons butter

### Other

- 2 tablespoons cooking spray for greasing the waffle maker
- 2 tablespoons freshly chopped parsley

## Directions:

1. Preheat the waffle maker.
2. Add the eggs, grated mozzarella cheese, almond flour, coconut flour and baking powder to a bowl and season with salt and pepper.
3. Mix until just combined.
4. Spray the waffle maker with cooking spray to prevent the chaffles from sticking. Add a few tablespoons of the batter to the heated and greased waffle maker.
5. Close the lid and cook for about 7 minutes depending on your waffle maker.
6. Repeat with the rest of the batter.
7. Meanwhile, melt the butter in a nonstick pan over medium heat.
8. Season the chicken with salt and pepper and dried oregano and mix in the minced garlic.
9. Cook the chicken for about 10 minutes, stirring constantly.
10. Serve each chaffle with a topping of the garlic chicken mixture and sprinkle some freshly chopped parsley on top.

## Nutrition:

Calories 475, fat 29.5 g, carbs 7.2 g, sugar 0.4 g, Protein 44.7 g, sodium 286 mg

# Chicken Taco Chaffle

Preparation time: 10 minutes

Cooking Time:15 Minutes

Servings: 2

## Ingredients:

### Batter

- 4 eggs
- 2 cups grated provolone cheese
- 6 tablespoons almond flour
- 2½ teaspoons baking powder
- Salt and pepper to taste

### Chicken topping

- 2 tablespoons olive oil
- ½ pound ground chicken
- Salt and pepper to taste
- 1 garlic clove, minced
- 2 teaspoons dried oregano

## Other

- 2 tablespoons butter to brush the waffle maker
- 2 tablespoons freshly chopped spring onion for garnishing

## Directions:

1. Preheat the waffle maker.
2. Add the eggs, grated provolone cheese, almond flour, baking powder and salt and pepper to a bowl.
3. Mix until just combined.
4. Brush the heated waffle maker with cooking spray and add a few tablespoons of the batter.
5. Close the lid and cook for about 7–9 minutes depending on your waffle maker.
6. Meanwhile, heat the olive oil in a nonstick pan over medium heat and start cooking the ground chicken.
7. Season with salt and pepper and stir in the minced garlic and dried oregano. Cook for 10 minutes.
8. Add some of the cooked ground chicken to each chaffle and serve with freshly chopped spring onion.

**Nutrition:** Calories 584, fat 44 g, carbs 6.4 g, sugar 0.8 g, Protein 41.3g, sodium 737 mg

# Italian Chicken and Basil Chaffle

Preparation time: 10 minutes

Cooking Time:7–9 Minutes

Servings: 2

## Ingredients:

### Batter

- ½ pound ground chicken
- 4 eggs
- 3 tablespoons tomato sauce
- Salt and pepper to taste
- 1 cup grated mozzarella cheese
- 1 teaspoon dried oregano
- 3 tablespoons freshly chopped basil leaves
- ½ teaspoon dried garlic

### Other

- 2 tablespoons butter to brush the waffle maker
- ¼ cup tomato sauce for serving
- 1 tablespoon freshly chopped basil for serving

## Directions:

1. Preheat the waffle maker.
2. Add the ground chicken, eggs and tomato sauce to a bowl and season with salt and pepper.
3. Add the mozzarella cheese and season with dried oregano, freshly chopped basil and dried garlic.
4. Mix until fully combined and batter forms.
5. Brush the heated waffle maker with butter and add a few tablespoons of the chaffle batter.
6. Close the lid and cook for about 7–9 minutes depending on your waffle maker.
7. Repeat with the rest of the batter.
8. Serve with tomato sauce and freshly chopped basil on top.

## Nutrition:

Calories 250, fat 15.7 g, carbs 2.5 g, sugar 1.5 g, Protein 24.5 g, sodium 334 mg

# Beef Meatballs on A Chaffle

Preparation time: 10 minutes

Cooking Time:20 Minutes

Servings: 2

## Ingredients:

**Batter**

- 4 eggs
- 2½ cups grated gouda cheese
- ¼ cup heavy cream
- Salt and pepper to taste
- 1 spring onion, finely chopped
- Beef meatballs
- 1 pound ground beef
- Salt and pepper to taste
- 2 teaspoons Dijon mustard
- 1 spring onion, finely chopped
- 5 tablespoons almond flour
- 2 tablespoons butter

## Other

- 2 tablespoons cooking spray to brush the waffle maker
- 2 tablespoons freshly chopped parsley

## Directions:

1. Preheat the waffle maker.
2. Add the eggs, grated gouda cheese, heavy cream, salt and pepper and finely chopped spring onion to a bowl.
3. Mix until combined and batter forms.
4. Brush the heated waffle maker with cooking spray and add a few tablespoons of the batter.
5. Close the lid and cook for about 7 minutes depending on your waffle maker.
6. Meanwhile, mix the ground beef meat, salt and pepper, Dijon mustard, chopped spring onion and almond flour in a large bowl.
7. Form small meatballs with your hands.
8. Heat the butter in a nonstick frying pan and cook the beef meatballs for about 3–4 minutes on each side.
9. Serve each chaffle with a couple of meatballs and some freshly chopped parsley on top.

**Nutrition:** Calories 670, fat 47.4g, carbs 4.6 g, sugar 1.7 g, Protein 54.9 g, sodium 622 mg

# Leftover Turkey Chaffle

Preparation time: 10 minutes

Cooking Time:7–9 Minutes

Servings: 2

**Ingredients:**

**Batter**

- ½ pound shredded leftover turkey meat
- 4 eggs
- 1 cup grated provolone cheese
- Salt and pepper to taste
- 1 teaspoon dried basil
- ½ teaspoon dried garlic
- 3 tablespoons sour cream
- 2 tablespoons coconut flour

**Other**

- 2 tablespoons cooking spray for greasing the chaffle maker
- ¼ cup cream cheese for serving the chaffles

## Directions:

1. Preheat the waffle maker.
2. Add the leftover turkey, eggs and provolone cheese to a bowl and season with salt and pepper, dried basil and dried garlic.
3. Add the sour cream and coconut flour and mix until batter forms.
4. Brush the heated waffle maker with cooking spray and add a few tablespoons of the chaffle batter.
5. Close the lid and cook for about 7–9 minutes depending on your waffle maker.
6. Repeat with the rest of the batter.
7. Serve with cream cheese on top of each chaffle.

## Nutrition:

Calories 372, fat 27.g, carbs 5.4 g, sugar 0.6 g, Protein 25 g, sodium 795 mg

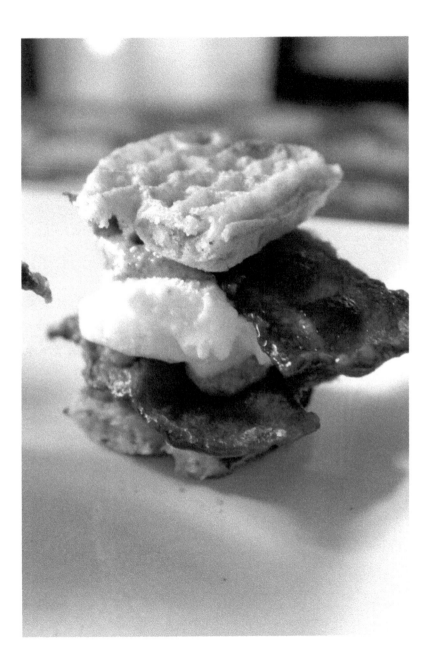

Lightning Source UK Ltd.
Milton Keynes UK
UKHW021844040521
383144UK00003B/374

9 781802 771541